I0048417

Blood Chemistry and CBC Analysis —
Clinical Laboratory Testing from a Functional Perspective

Quick Reference Guide

Dicken Weatherby, N.D.
Scott Ferguson, N.D.

Bear Mountain Publishing • Jacksonville, OR

Blood Chemistry and CBC Analysis- Clinical Laboratory Testing from a Functional Perspective
Quick Reference Guide

© 2005 By Weatherby & Associates, LLC
All rights reserved. No part of this book may be reproduced or transmitted in any form or by any means, electronic or mechanical, including photocopying, recording, or by any information storage or retrieval system without written permission from the authors, except for the inclusion of quotations in a review.

Bear Mountain Publishing
1-541-899-1522

ISBN: 0-9761367-8-3

Warning - Disclaimer
Bear Mountain Publishing has designed this book to provide information in regard to the subject matter covered. It is sold with the understanding that the publisher and the authors are not liable for the misconception or misuse of information provided. The purpose of this book is to educate. It is not meant to be a comprehensive source for blood chemistry and CBC analysis, and is not intended as a substitute for medical diagnosis or treatment, or intended as a substitute for medical counseling. Information contained in this book should not be construed as a claim or representation that any treatment, process or interpretation mentioned constitutes a cure, palliative, or ameliorative. The interpretation is intended to supplement the practitioner's knowledge of their patient. It should be considered as adjunctive support to other diagnostic medical procedures.

Printed in the United States of America

How to Order
For mail orders call in the United States at 541-899-1522 or online at www.BloodChemistryAnalysis.com

Introduction

There are few diagnostic tests that are truly diagnostic all on their own. It is important to see the trends and patterns that exist between various tests. This section is organized to provide that information, and is broken into two sections.

Section One

The first section of the Quick Reference Guide is a list of the individual components of the blood chemistry screen and complete blood count. Beside each component, organized by high or low values, is a list of the most common conditions seen with deviations from normal.

COMPONENT	HIGH	LOW
Glucose	• Insulin resistance • Early stage hyperglycemia/Diabetes • Syndrome X/Metabolic Syndrome • Thiamine Need • Cortisol resistance • Fatty liver • Liver congestion	• Hypoglycemia- reactive • Hypoglycemia- Liver glycogen problem • Hyperinsulinism • Adrenal hypofunction
Hemoglobin A1C	• Diabetes mellitus • Insulin resistance	• Hypoglycemia
Triglycerides	• Syndrome X/Metabolic Syndrome • Fatty liver • Liver congestion • Insulin resistance • Cardiovascular disease • Atherosclerosis • Poor metabolism and utilization of fats • Early stage hyperglycemia/Diabetes • Hyperlipidemia/ Hyperlipoproteinemia • Primary hypothyroidism • Adrenal cortical dysfunction • Secondary hypothyroidism- anterior pituitary dysfunction • Alcoholism	• Liver/biliary dysfunction • Thyroid hyperfunction • Autoimmune processes • Adrenal hyperfunction

COMPONENT	HIGH	LOW
Cholesterol	• Primary hypothyroidism • Adrenal cortical dysfunction • Cardiovascular disease • Atherosclerosis • Biliary stasis • Insulin resistance • Poor metabolism and utilization of fats • Fatty liver • Early stage hyperglycemia/Diabetes • Syndrome X/Metabolic Syndrome • Hyperlipoproteinemia • Multiple sclerosis	• Oxidative stress • Heavy metal body burden • Liver/biliary dysfunction • Diet- malnutrition • Thyroid hyperfunction • Autoimmune processes • Adrenal hyperfunction
LDL		• Diet- high in refined carbohydrates • Syndrome X/Metabolic Syndrome • Atherosclerosis • Fatty liver/Hyperlipidemia • Oxidative stress
HDL	• Autoimmune processes	• Hyperlipidemia/Fatty Liver • Atherosclerosis • Syndrome X/Metabolic Syndrome • Oxidative stress • Heavy metals • Hyperthyroidism • Lack of exercise/sedentary lifestyle
BUN	• Renal disease • Renal insufficiency • Dehydration • Hypochlorhydria • Diet- excessive protein intake • Adrenal hyperfunction • Dysbiosis • Edema • Anterior pituitary dysfunction	• Diet- low protein • Malabsorption • Pancreatic insufficiency • Liver dysfunction

© Weatherby & Associates, LLC

COMPONENT	HIGH	LOW
Creatinine	• BPH • Urinary tract congestion • Renal disease • Renal insufficiency • Uterine hypertrophy	• Muscle atrophy • Protein insufficiency or impaired digestion
Bun/Creatinine ratio	• Renal disease	• Diet- low protein • Posterior pituitary dysfunction
Uric Acid	• Gout • Atherosclerosis/Oxidative stress • Arthralgias • Renal insufficiency/Renal disease • Circulatory disorders • Leaky gut syndrome	• Molybdenum deficiency • Anemia- B12/folate deficiency • Copper deficiency
Potassium	• Adrenal hypofunction • Dehydration • Tissue destruction • Metabolic acidosis	• Adrenal hyperfunction • Drug diuretics • Benign essential hypertension
Sodium	• Adrenal hyperfunction • Cushing's disease • Dehydration	• Adrenal hypofunction • Addison's disease • Edema • Drug diuretics
Chloride	• Metabolic acidosis • Adrenal hyperfunction	• Hypochlorhydria • Metabolic alkalosis • Adrenal hypofunction
CO2	• Metabolic alkalosis • Adrenal hyperfunction • Hypochlorhydria • Respiratory acidosis	• Metabolic acidosis • Thiamine need • Respiratory alkalosis
Anion Gap	• Thiamine need • Metabolic acidosis	
Total Protein	• Dehydration	• Hypochlorhydria • Digestive dysfunction and/or inflammation • Liver dysfunction

COMPONENT	HIGH	LOW
Albumin	• Dehydration	• Hypochlorhydria • Liver dysfunction • Oxidative stress • Vitamin C need
Globulin	• Hypochlorhydria • Liver cell damage • Oxidative stress • Heavy metal toxicity	• Digestive dysfunction and/or inflammation • Immune insufficiency
Albumin/ Globulin ratio		• Liver dysfunction • Immune activation
Calcium	• Parathyroid hyperfunction • Thyroid hypofunction • Impaired membrane health	• Parathyroid hypofunction • Calcium need • Hypochlorhydria
Phosphorous	• Parathyroid hypofunction • Bone growth and/or repair • Diet- excessive phosphorous consumption • Renal insufficiency	• Parathyroid hyperfunction • Hypochlorhydria • Hyperinsulinism • Diet- high in refined carbohydrates
Magnesium	• Renal dysfunction • Thyroid hypofunction	• Epilepsy • Muscle spasm
Alkaline phosphatase	• Biliary obstruction • Liver cell damage • Bone: loss/increased turnover or bone growth and/or repair • Leaky gut syndrome • Herpes zoster • Metastatic carcinoma of the bone	• Zinc deficiency
LDH	• Liver/biliary dysfunction • Cardiovascular disease • Anemia- B12/folate deficiency, hemolytic • Non-specific tissue inflammation • Tissue destruction • Viral infection	• Reactive hypoglycemia

COMPONENT	HIGH	LOW
SGOT/AST	• Dysfunction located outside of the liver and Biliary tree • Developing Congestive Heart Failure • Acute MI • Cardiovascular dysfunction: Coronary artery insufficiency • Liver cell damage • Liver dysfunction • Excess muscle breakdown or turnover • Infectious mononucleosis, EBV, CMV	• B6 deficiency • Alcoholism
SGPT/ALT	• Dysfunction located in the liver • Fatty liver • Liver dysfunction • Biliary tract obstruction • Excessive muscle breakdown or turnover • Cirrhosis of the liver • Liver cell damage	• B6 deficiency • Fatty liver (early development) • Liver congestion • Alcoholism
GGTP	• Dysfunction located outside the liver and inside the biliary tree • Biliary obstruction • Biliary stasis/insufficiency • Liver cell damage • Alcoholism • Acute/chronic Pancreatitis • Pancreatic insufficiency	• B6 deficiency • Magnesium need
Total Bilirubin	• Biliary stasis • Oxidative stress • Thymus dysfunction • Biliary tract obstruction or calculi • Liver dysfunction • RBC hemolysis • Gilbert's syndrome	• Spleen insufficiency

© Weatherby & Associates, LLC

www.BloodChemistryAnalysis.com

COMPONENT	HIGH	LOW
Direct Bilirubin	• Biliary tract obstruction • Biliary calculi/obstruction (usually extra hepatic)	
Indirect Bilirubin	• RBC hemolysis • Gilbert's syndrome	
Serum Iron	• Liver dysfunction • Hemochromatosis/hemosiderosis/iron overload • Iron conversion problem • Viral infection • Excess iron consumption	• Anemia- iron deficiency • Hypochlorhydria • Internal/microscopic bleeding
Ferritin	• Hemochromatosis/hemosiderosis/iron overload • Excess iron consumption • Inflammation/liver dysfunction/oxidative stress	• Anemia- iron deficiency
TIBC	• Anemia- iron deficiency • Internal bleeding	• Hemochromatosis/hemosiderosis/iron overload • Microscopic bleeding • Diet- protein malnutrition
% Transferrin Saturation	• Hemochromatosis/hemosiderosis/iron overload	• Anemia- iron deficiency
TSH	• Primary hypothyroidism	• Hyperthyroidism • Secondary hypothyroidism- anterior pituitary dysfunction • Tertiary hypothyroidism- hypothalamic dysfunction • Heavy metal body burden
T-3	• Hyperthyroidism • Iodine deficiency	• Primary hypothyroidism • Selenium deficiency
T-4	• Hyperthyroidism • Thyroid hormone replacement	• Primary hypothyroidism • Iodine deficiency
T-3 Uptake	• Hyperthyroidism • Thyroid hormone replacement	• Primary hypothyroidism • Secondary hypothyroidism- anterior pituitary dysfunction • Selenium deficiency • Iodine deficiency
ESR	• Non-specific tissue inflammation or destruction	

© Weatherby & Associates, LLC

COMPLETE BLOOD COUNT

COMPONENT	HIGH/LOW	CONDITION
White Blood Cell Count	• Childhood diseases (Measles, Mumps, Rubella, Chicken pox etc.) • Acute bacterial infection • Acute viral infection • Stress • Diet- High in refined carbohydrates	• Chronic viral infections • Chronic bacterial infections • Leukocytic auto-digestion • Systemic Lupus Erythematosis (SLE) • Decreased production from bone marrow • Diet- raw food diet
Red Blood Cell Count	• Respiratory distress: Asthma or emphysema • Polycythemia (relative or absolute) • Dehydration	• Anemia- Iron deficiency • Anemia- B12/folate deficiency • Anemia- Copper deficiency • Internal bleeding • Vitamin C need
Hemoglobin	• Respiratory distress: Asthma or emphysema • Polycythemia (relative or primary) • Dehydration	• Anemia- iron deficiency • Anemia- B12/folate deficiency • Anemia- B6 deficiency anemia • Anemia- Copper deficiency • Internal bleeding • Digestive inflammation • Vitamin C need
Hematocrit	• Respiratory distress: Asthma or emphysema • Polycythemia (relative or primary) • Spleen hyperfunction • Dehydration	• Anemia • Anemia- Iron deficiency • Anemia- B12/folate deficiency • Anemia- B6 deficiency • Anemia- Copper deficiency • Internal bleeding • Digestive inflammation • Thymus hypofunction • Vitamin C need
MCV	• Anemia- B12/folate deficiency • Vitamin C need	• Anemia- Iron deficiency • Anemia- B6 deficiency • Internal bleeding

© Weatherby & Associates, LLC

www.BloodChemistryAnalysis.com

COMPONENT	HIGH	LOW
MCH	• Anemia- B12/folate deficiency • Hypochlorhydria	• Anemia- Iron deficiency • Anemia- B6 deficiency • Internal bleeding • Heavy metal body burden • Vitamin C need
MCHC	• Anemia- B12/folate deficiency • Hypochlorhydria	• Anemia- Iron deficiency • Anemia- B6 deficiency • Heavy metal body burden • Vitamin C need
RDW	• Anemia- Iron deficiency • Anemia- B12/folate deficiency • Pernicious anemia	• Childhood diseases (Measles, Mumps, Rubella, Chicken pox) • Acute or chronic bacterial infection • Inflammation
Neutrophils		• Blood diseases (aplastic anemia, pernicious anemia etc.) • Chronic viral infection
Monocytes	• Recovery phase of infection • Liver dysfunction • Intestinal parasites • Benign Prostatic Hypertrophy (BPH)	
Lymphocytes	• Childhood diseases • Acute and chronic viral infection • Infectious mononucleosis • Inflammation • Systemic toxicity	• Chronic viral or bacterial infections • Free radical activity • Active bacterial infection • Suppressed bone marrow function
Eosinophils	• Intestinal parasites • Food and environmental allergies/sensitivities • Asthma	• Increased adrenal steroid production
Basophils	• Tissue inflammation • Intestinal parasites	
Platelet count	• Atherosclerosis	• Idiopathic thrombocytopenia • Heavy metal body burden • Free radical pathology

© Weatherby & Associates, LLC

Section Two

The second section presents the common patterns arranged by conditions. Beside each condition is a list of the patterns organized by which components of the blood chemistry screen and complete blood count are high or low for any given condition. The optimal value changes are given for both the Standard US Units and Standard International Units.

CONDITION	HIGH	LOW
Adrenal hyperfunction	↑ Sodium (>142) ↑ Chloride (>106) ↑ CO2 (>30) ↑ BUN (>16 or 5.71 mmol/L)	↓ Potassium (<4.0) ↓ Cholesterol (<150 or 3.9mmol/L) ↓ Triglyceride (<70 or 0.79mmol/L)
Adrenal hypofunction	↑ Potassium (>4.5) ↑ Cholesterol (>220 or 5.69mmol/L) ↑ Triglycerides (>110 or 1.24 mmol/L)	↓ Sodium (<135) ↓ Chloride (<100) ↓ Blood Glucose (<80 or 4.44 mol/L)
Anemia- B12/folate deficiency	↑ MCH (>31.9) ↑ MCV (>89.9) ↑ RDW (>13) ↑ MCHC (>35) ↑ Serum iron (>100 or >17.91 μmol/L) ↑ LDH (>200)	↓ RBCs (<3.9♀, <4.2♂) ↓ HCT (<37 or 0.37 in ♂ and <40 or 0.4 in ♂) ↓ HGB (<13.5 or 135g/L in ♀ and <14 or 140 in ♂) ↓ WBCs (<5.0) ↓Neutrophils (<40) ↓ Uric acid (<3.5 or 208 μmol/dL)
Anemia- hemolytic	↑ LDH (>200) ↑ Reticulocytes (>1 or 00.1)	
Anemia- Iron deficiency	↑ TIBC (>350) ↑ Transferrin **If hypochlorhydria is present:** ↑ Globulin (>2.8 or 28 g/L)	↓ Serum iron (<50 or <8.96 μmol/L) ↓ Ferritin (<10 in ♀ and <33 in ♂) ↓ % transferrin saturation (<20%) ↓ or N RBCs (<3.9♀, <4.2♂) ↓ HGB (<13.5 or 135 g/L in ♂ and <14 or140 in ♂) ↓ or N HCT (<37 or 0.37 in ♂ and <40 or 0.4 in ♂) ↓ MCV MCV (<82), ↓ MCH (<28), ↓ MCHC (<32) ↓ Globulin (<2.4 or 24 g/L) ↓ Phosphorous (<3.0 or 0.97 mmol/L)
Anterior pituitary/secondary thyroid hypofunction	↑ Triglycerides (>110 or 1.24 mmol/L) ↑ Cholesterol (>220 or 5.69mmol/L) ↑ BUN (>16 or 5.71 mmol/L)	↓TSH (<2.0) ↓ T-3 uptake (<27)

© Weatherby & Associates, LLC

www.BloodChemistryAnalysis.com

CONDITION	HIGH	LOW
Arthralgias	↑ ESR (> 10 in ♀ and > 5 in ♂) ↑ C-reactive protein ↑ or **N** albumin (>5.0 or 50 g/L) ↑ Globulin (>2.8 or 28 g/L) ↑ Platelet (>385)	↓ or **N** albumin (<4.0 or 40 g/L)
Asthma	↑ HGB (>14.5 or 145 g/L in ♂ and >15 or 150 in ♂) ↑ Eosinophils (>3%) ↑ HCT (>44 or 0.44 in ♂ and >48 or 0.48 in ♂) ↑ Neutrophils (>60%) ↑ or **N** Total WBC (>7.5)	↓ Lymphocytes ↓ Plasma and salivary cortisol in the chronic phase.
Atherosclerosis	↑ Triglycerides (>110 or 1.24 mmol/L) ↑ or **N** Cholesterol (>220 or 5.69mmol/L) ↑ LDL (>120 or 3.1 mmol/L) ↑ Uric acid (>5.9 or 351 μmol/dL) ↑ Platelet (>385) ↑ C reactive protein	↓ HDL (<55 or 1.42 mmol/L)
Autoimmune processes- tissue destruction	↑ HDL (>70 or 1.81 mmol/L) ↑ LDH (>200)	↓ Triglyceride (<70 or 0.79 mmol/L) ↓ or **N** Cholesterol (<150 or 3.9 mmol/L)
B6 deficiency (confirm with a serum or urinary homocysteine)	**N** Serum iron	↓ or **N** SGPT/ALT (<10) ↓ SGOT/AST (<10) ↓ GGTP (<10) ↓ MCV (<82), ↓ MCH (<28) ↓ MCHC (<32) ↓ HCT (<37 or 0.37 in ♂ and <40 or 0.4 in ♂) ↓ HGB (<13.5 or 135 g/L in ♂ and <14 or 140 in ♂)
Biliary dysfunction	↑ Alkaline phosphatase (>100) ↑ GGTP (>30) ↑ SGPT/ALT (>30) ↑ LDH (>200)	↓ Triglyceride (<70 or 0.79 mmol/L) ↓ Cholesterol (<150 or 3.9 mmol/L)
Biliary obstruction/calculi	↑ Alkaline phosphatase (>100) ↑ SGPT/ALT (>30) ↑ GGTP (>30) ↑ Bilirubin (>1.2 or 20.5 μmol/dL) ↑ Direct bilirubin (>0.2 or 3.4 μmol/dL)	

© Weatherby & Associates, LLC

www.BloodChemistryAnalysis.com

CONDITION	HIGH	LOW
Biliary stasis/insufficiency	↑ Cholesterol (>220 or 5.69 mmol/L) ↑ GGTP (>30) ↑ Bilirubin (>1.2 or 20.5 μmol/dL) ↑ Alk Phos (>100)	
BPH	↑ Creatinine (>1.1 or 97.2 mmol/L) ↑ PSA (may be normal) ↑ Monocytes (>7%)	
Cardiovascular disease	↑ Triglycerides (>110 or 1.24 mmol/L) ↑ Cholesterol (>220 or 5.69mmol/L) ↑ LDL (>120 or 3.1 mmol/L) ↑ LDH (>200) ↑ SGOT/AST (>30)	↓ HDL (<55 or 1.42 mmol/L)
Childhood diseases	↑ Total WBC (>7.5) ↑ Neutrophils (>60%) (early) ↑ Lymphocytes (>44%)(later)	↓ Neutrophils (<40%) (later) ↓ Lymphocytes (<24%) (early)
Copper deficiency	Low high MCV (>89.9) ↑ to N MCH (>31.9),	↓ Uric acid (<3.5 or 208 μmol/dL) ↓ HCT (<37 or 0.37 in ♂ and <40 or 0.4 in ♂) ↓ HGB (<13.5 or 135 g/L in ♂ and <14 or 140 in ♂) ↓ RBCs (<3.9♀, <4.2♂)
Deficient Red Blood Cell production	↑ Serum iron (>100 or >17.91 μmol/L)	↓ RBCs (<3.9♀, <4.2♂) ↓ HCT (<37 or 0.37 in ♂ and <40 or 0.4 in ♂)
Dehydration	↑ RBCs (>4.5 in ♂ and >4.9 in ♂) ↑ HGB (>14.5 or 145 g/L in ♂ and >15 or 150 in ♂) ↑ HCT (>44 or 0.44 in ♂ and >48 or 0.48 in ♂) ↑ Total protein (> 7.4 or 74 g/L) (Chronic) ↑ Albumin (>5.0 or 50 g/L) (Chronic) ↑ Sodium (>142) ↑ Potassium (<4.0) ↑ BUN (>16 or 5.71 mmol/L) (Chronic)	
Diabetes/hyperglycemia	↑ Blood Glucose (>100 or 5.55 mmol/L) ↑ Hemoglobin A1C (>5.7% or 0.057) ↑ Cholesterol (>220 or 5.69 mmol/L) ↑ Triglycerides (>110 or 1.24 mmol/L) ↑ BUN (>16 or 5.71 mmol/L) ↑ Creatinine (>1.1 or 97.2 μmmol/dL)	↓ HDL (<55 or 1.42 mmol/L)

© Weatherby & Associates, LLC

CONDITION	HIGH	LOW
Diet- fat deficient		↓ Cholesterol (<150 or 3.9mmol/L) ↓ Triglyceride (<70 or 0.79mmol/L)
Diet- high in refined carbohydrates	↑ LDL (>120 or 3.1 mmol/L)	↓ Phosphorous (<3.0 or 0.97 mmol/L) ↓ Total WBC count (<5.0)
Diet- low protein		↓ BUN (<10 or 3.57 mmol/L) ↓ Total protein (< 6.9 or 69 g/L) ↓ BUN-Creatinine ratio (<13) ↓ Creatinine (<0.8 or 70.7 μmol/dL)
Digestive dysfunction/inflammation	↑ BUN (>16 or 5.71 mmol/L) ↑ Basophils (>1%) **With Ulceration or erosion:** ↑ Alk Phos intestinal isoenzyme	↓ Total protein (< 6.9 or 69 g/L) ↓ Total Globulin (<2.4 or 24 g/L) ↓ Albumin (<4.0 or 40 g/L) ↓ Phosphorous (<3.0 or 0.97 mmol/L) ↓ Creatinine (<0.8 or 70.7 μmol/dL)
Edema	↑ BUN (>16 or 5.71 mmol/L)	↓ Sodium (<135) ↓ albumin (<4.0 or 40 g/L)
Emphysema	↑ HCT (>44 or 0.44 in ♂ and >48 or 0.48 in ♂) ↑ RBCs (>4.5 in ♂ and >4.9 in ♂) ↑ or **N** CO_2 (>30)	↓↓ Alpha I globulin ↓ or **N** serum chloride (<100)
Excess consumption of iron	↑ Serum iron (>100 or >17.91 μmol/L) ↑ Ferritin (>122 in ♂ and >236 in ♂)	
Fatty Liver (steatosis)	↑ SGPT/ALT (>30) ↑ LDH (>200) ↑ Alk Phos (>100)	
Fatty liver- Early Stage	↑ Blood Glucose (>100 or 5.55 mmol/L) ↑ Triglycerides (>110 or 1.24 mmol/L) ↑ Cholesterol (>220 or 5.69mmol/L) ↑ LDL (>120 or 3.1 mmol/L)	↓ HDL (<55 or 1.42 mmol/L) ↓ SGPT/ALT (<10)
Gilbert's syndrome	↑ Bilirubin (>1.2 or 20.5 μmol/dL) ↑ Indirect bilirubin (>1.0 or 17.1 μmol/dL)	
Gout	↑↑ Uric acid (>5.9 or 351 μmol/dL) ↑ Cholesterol (>220 or 5.69mmol/L) ↑ BUN (>16 or 5.71 mmol/L) ↑ or **N** Creatinine (>1.1 or 97.2 μmmol/dL)	↓ Phosphorous (<3.0 or 0.97 mmol/L)

© Weatherby & Associates, LLC

CONDITION	HIGH	LOW
Heavy metal burden (run a hair/urine analysis if this pattern comes up to rule this out)	↑ Uric acid (>5.9 or 351 μmol/dL) ↑ Total Bilirubin (>1.2 or 20.5 μmol/dL) ↑ BUN (>16 or 5.71 mmol/L) **Cadmium toxicity:** ↑ Calcium (>10.5 or 2.5 mmol/L)	↓ MCHC (<32) and MCH (<28) ↓ HCT (<37 or 0.37 in ♂ and <40 or 0.4 in ♂) ↓ HGB (<13.5 or 135 g/L in ♂ and <14 or 140 in ♂) ↓ RBCs (<3.9♀, <4.2♂) ↓ 5th Isoenzyme of LDH **Cadmium toxicity:** ↓ Phosphorous (<3.0 or 0.97 mmol/L)
Heavy metals/chemical toxicity	↑ Total globulin (>2.8 or 28 g/L)	↓ Uric acid (<3.5 or 208 μmmol/L) ↓ Cholesterol (<150 or 3.9mmol/L) ↓ HDL (<55 or 1.42 mmol/L) ↓ MCH (<28) ↓ MCHC (<32) ↓ TSH (<2.0) ↓ Platelets (<155)
Hemochromatosis	↑ Serum iron (>100 or >17.91 μmol/L) ↑↑ Ferritin (>1000) ↑ % transferrin saturation (>35%) ↑ SGOT/AST (>30)	↓ TIBC (<250 or 44.8 μmol/dL)
Hyperinsulinemia	↑ Triglycerides (>110 or 1.24 mmol/L) ↑ Cholesterol (>220 or 5.69mmol/L)	↓ Blood Glucose (<80 or 4.44 mol/L) ↓ HDL (<55 or 1.42 mmol/L) ↓ Phosphorous (<3.0 or 0.97 mmol/L)
Hyperlipidemia	↑ Triglycerides (>110 or 1.24 mmol/L) ↑ Cholesterol (>220 or 5.69mmol/L) ↑ LDL (>120 or 3.1 mmol/L)	↓ HDL (<55 or 1.42 mmol/L)
Hyperlipoproteinemia	↑ Triglycerides (>110 or 1.24 mmol/L) ↑ Cholesterol (>220 or 5.69mmol/L)	
Hypochlorhydria	↑ BUN (>16 or 5.71 mmol/L) ↑ Total Globulin (>2.8 or 28 g/L)	↓ or **N** Total protein (< 6.9 or 69 g/L) ↓ or **N** albumin (<4.0 or 40 g/L) ↓ Phosphorous (<3.0 or 0.97 mmol/L)
Hypoglycemia- liver glycogen storage problem	↑ SGPT/ALT (>30)	↓ Blood Glucose (<80 or 4.44 mol/L) ↓ Hemoglobin A1C (<4.1% or 0.041) ↓ LDH (<140)

© Weatherby & Associates, LLC

www.BloodChemistryAnalysis.com

CONDITION	HIGH	LOW
Hypoglycemia-reactive		↓ Blood Glucose (<80 or 4.44 mol/L) ↓ Hemoglobin A1C (<4.1% or 0.041) ↓ LDH (<140)
Increased Red blood cell destruction	↑ Bilirubin (>1.2 or 20.5 μmol/dL) ↑ Indirect bilirubin (>1.0 or 17.1 μmol/dL)	↓ RBCs (<3.9♀, <4.2♂)
Infection: active	↑ Total WBC (>7.5) ↑ Neutrophils (>60%) ↑ Bands (>5%) ↑ ESR (> 10 in ♀ and > 5 in ♂)	↓ Lymphocytes (<24%)
Infection: Acute bacterial	↑ WBCs ↑ Neutrophils (>60%) ↑ Monocytes (recovery phase) (>7%) ↑ Bands (>5%) ↑ ESR (> 10 in ♀ and > 5 in ♂)	↓ or N Lymphocytes (<24%)
Infection: Acute viral	↑ Total WBC (>7.5) ↑ Lymphocytes (>44%) ↑ Monocytes (>7%) (recovery phase) ↑ Bands (>5%) ↑ ESR (> 10 in ♀ and > 5 in ♂) ↑ LDH (>200)	↓ or N Neutrophils (<40%)
Infection: Chronic viral	↑ Serum iron (>100 or >17.91 μmol/L)	↓ Total WBC count (<5.0) ↓ Lymphocytes (<24%)
Inflammation- non-specific	↑ LDH (>200) ↑ ESR (> 10 in ♀ and > 5 in ♂) ↑ Ferritin (>122 in ♂ and >236 in ♂) ↑ Basophils (>1%)	
Insulin Resistance	↑ Blood Glucose (>100 or 5.55 mmol/L) ↑ Hemoglobin A1C (>5.7% or 0.057) ↑ Triglycerides (>110 or 1.24 mmol/L) ↑ Cholesterol (>220 or 5.69mmol/L)	
Internal bleeding	↑ Reticulocyte count (>1%) ↑ TIBC (>350 or 62.7 μmol/dL) ↑ Transferrin.	↓ or N Serum iron (<50 or <8.96 μmol/L) ↓ or N serum Ferritin (<10 in ♀ and <33 in ♂) ↓ HGB (<13.5 or 135 g/L in ♂ and <14 or 140 in ♂) ↓ or N HCT (<37 or 0.37 in ♂ and <40 or 0.4 in ♂) ↓ MCV (<89.9), ↓ MCH (<28)

© Weatherby & Associates, LLC

www.BloodChemistryAnalysis.com

CONDITION	HIGH	LOW
Internal microscopic bleeding	↑ Reticulocyte count (>1%)	↓ TIBC (<250 or 44.8 μmol/dL) ↓ Transferrin
Intestinal parasites	↑ Eosinophils (>3%) ↑ or **N** Basophils (>1%) ↑ or **N** Monocytes (>7%) ↑ IgE Stool positive for parasites or ova	↓ or **N** Serum iron (<50 or <8.96 μmol/L) ↓/**N** HGB (<13.5 or 135 g/L in ♂ & <14 or 140 in ♂) ↓ or **N** HCT (<37 or 0.37 in ♂ and <40 or 0.4 in ♂)
Iodine deficiency	↑ T-3 (>230 or 3.53 nmol/L)	↓ T-3 uptake (<27) ↓ T-4 (<6 or 7.2 nmol/L)
Leaky gut syndrome	↑ Uric acid (>5.9 or 351 μmol/dL) ↑ Alkaline phosphatase (>100)	
Liver cell damage	↑ Globulin (>2.8 or 28 g/L) ↑ Alkaline phosphatase (>100) ↑ SGOT/AST (>30) ↑ SGPT/ALT (>30) ↑ GGTP (>30)	
Liver dysfunction	↑ SGPT/ALT (>30) ↑ LDH (>200) ↑ SGOT/AST (>30) ↑ Bilirubin (>1.2 or 20.5 μmol/dL) ↑ Direct bilirubin (>0.2 or 3.4 μmol/dL) ↑ Serum iron (>100 or >17.91 μmol/L) ↑ Ferritin (>122 in ♂ and >236 in ♂) ↑ Monocytes (>7%)	↓ BUN (<10 or 3.57 mmol/L) ↓ Total protein (< 6.9 or 69 g/L) ↓ Albumin (<4.0 or 40 g/L) ↓ Albumin/globulin ratio ↓ Triglyceride (<70 or 0.79mmol/L) ↓ Cholesterol (<150 or 3.9mmol/L)
Malabsorption		↓ BUN (<10 or 3.57 mmol/L) ↓ GGTP (<10)
Metabolic acidosis	↑ Chloride (>106) ↑ Anion gap (>12) ↑ Potassium (>4.5)	↓ CO2 (<25)
Metabolic alkalosis	↑ CO2 (>30)	↓ Chloride (<100) ↓ Calcium (<9.2 or 2.3 mmol/L) ↓ Potassium (<4.0)
Microscopic bleeding	↑ Reticulocyte count (>1%)	↓ TIBC (<250 or 44.8 μmol/dL)

CONDITION	HIGH	LOW
Mononucleosis	↑ SGOT/AST (>30) ↑ Alkaline phosphatase (>100) ↑ LDH (>200) ↑ WBCs (2nd week) ↑ GGTP (>30) ↑ Lymphocytes (>44%)	↓ WBCs (1st week)
Muscle- atrophy or breakdown	↑ SGOT/AST (>30) ↑ SGPT/ALT (>30)	↓ Creatinine (<0.8 or 70.7 μmmol/dL)
Oxidative stress/Free radical activity	↑ LDL (>120 or 3.1 mmol/L) ↑ Uric acid (>5.9 or 351 μmol/dL) ↑ Total Globulin (>2.8 or 28 g/L) ↑ Bilirubin (>1.2 or 20.5 μmol/dL) ↑ Ferritin (>122 in ♂ and >236 in ♂)	↓ Lymphocytes (<24%) ↓ Cholesterol (below historical average) ↓ Albumin (<4.0 or 40 g/L) ↓ Platelets (<150)
Pancreatic insufficiency	↑ GGTP (>30)	↓ Total WBC count ↓ BUN (<10 or 3.57 mmol/L)
Parasites- intestinal	↑ Eosinophils (>3%) ↑ or **N** Basophils (>1%) ↑ or **N** Monocytes (>7%)	
Parathyroid hyperfunction	↑ Calcium (>10.5 or 2.5 mmol/L)	↓ Phosphorous (<3.0 or 0.97 mmol/L)
Parathyroid hypofunction	↑ Phosphorous (>4.0 or 1.29 mmol/L)	↓ Calcium (<9.2 or 2.3 mmol/L)
Polycythemia	↑ RBCs (>4.5 in ♂ and >4.9 in ♂) ↑ HCT (>44 or 0.44 in ♂ and >48 or 0.48 in ♂) ↑ HGB (>14.5 or 145 g/L in ♂ & >15 or 150 in ♂) ↑ Total Bilirubin (>1.2 or 20.5 μmol/dL) ↑ Uric acid (>5.9 or 351 μmol/dL) ↑ Total WBC (>7.5) ↑ Basophils (>1%) ↑ Alk phos (>100)	↓ or **N** MCV (<82) ↓ or **N** MCH (<28 ↓ or **N** Serum iron (<50 or <8.96 μmol/L)
Poor fat metabolism	↑ Triglycerides (>110 or 1.24 mmol/L) ↑ Cholesterol (>220 or 5.69 mmol/L)	
Posterior pituitary dysfunction		↓ BUN (<10 or 3.57 mmol/L) ↓ BUN-Creatinine ratio

© Weatherby & Associates, LLC

www.BloodChemistryAnalysis.com

CONDITION	HIGH	LOW
Pregnancy	↑ Total Cholesterol (>220 or 5.69mmol/L) ↑ MCV (>89.9) and MCH (>31.9) ↑ Neutrophils (>60%) ↑ T-4 (>12 or 154.4 nmol/L) ↑ Total WBC (>7.5) (late)	↓ Calcium in late pregnancy (<9.2 or 2.3 mmol/L) ↓ Albumin (<4.0 or 40 g/L) ↓ HGB (<13.5 or 135 g/L in ♂ and <14 or 140 in ♂) ↓ HCT (<37 or 0.37 in ♂ and <40 or 0.4 in ♂) ↓ T-3 uptake (<27) ↓ Lymphocytes (<24%) (late)) ↓ Total protein (< 6.9 or 69 g/L)
Renal insufficiency	↑ BUN (>16 or 5.71 mmol/L) ↑ or **N** Creatinine (>1.1 or 97.2 μmmol/dL) ↑ or **N** Uric acid (>5.9 or 351 μmol/dL) ↑ Phosphorous (>4.0 or 1.29 mmol/L	
Renal disease	↑ Creatinine (>1.1 or 97.2 μmmol/dL) ↑ BUN-Creatinine ratio ↑ BUN (>16 or 5.71 mmol/L) ↑ Uric acid (>5.9 or 351 μmol/dL) ↑ Phosphorous (>4.0 or 1.29 mmol/L ↑ LDH (>200) ↑ SGOT/AST (30)	
Respiratory distress	↑ RBCs (>4.5 in ♂ and >4.9 in ♂) ↑ HGB (>14.5 or 145 g/L in ♂ & >15 or 150 in ♂) ↑ HCT (>44 or 0.44 in ♂ and >48 or 0.48 in ♂) ↑ Eosinophils (>3%)	
Selenium deficiency		↓ T-3 (<100 or 1.54 nmol/L) ↓ T-3 uptake (<27)
Suppressed bone marrow production		↓ in all white blood cells ↓ RBCs (<3.9♀, <4.2♂) ↓ HCT (<37 or 0.37 in ♂ and <40 or 0.4 in ♂) ↓ HGB (<13.5 or 135 g/L in ♂ and <14 or 140 in ♂)
Syndrome X/Metabolic Syndrome	↑ Blood Glucose (>100 or 5.55 mmol/L) ↑ Triglycerides (>110 or 1.24 mmol/L) ↑ Cholesterol (>220 or 5.69mmol/L) ↑ LDL (>120 or 3.1 mmol/L) ↑ Hemoglobin A1C (>5.7% or 0.057)	↓ HDL (<55 or 1.42 mmol/L)
Systemic toxicity	↑ Lymphocytes (>44%)	

© Weatherby & Associates, LLC

www.BloodChemistryAnalysis.com

CONDITION	HIGH	LOW
Thiamine deficiency	↑ Blood Glucose (>100 or 5.55 mmol/L) ↑ Anion Gap (>12)	↓ CO2 (<26)
Thymus dysfunction	↑ Bilirubin (>1.2 or 20.5 μmol/dL) ↑ HGB (>14.5 or 145 g/L in ♂ and >15 or 150 in ♂) ↑ HCT (>44 or 0.44 in ♂ and >48 or 0.48 in ♂) ↑ RBCs (>4.5 in ♂ and >4.9 in ♂)	
Thyroid hormone replacement	↑ T-4 (>12 or 154.4 nmol/L) ↑ T-3 uptake (>37)	
Thyroid hyperfunction	↑ T-3 (>230 or 3.53 nmol/L) ↑ T-4 (>12 or 154.4 nmol/L) ↑ T-3 uptake (>37)	↓ Triglyceride (<70 or 0.79mmol/L) ↓ Cholesterol (<150 or 3.9mmol/L) ↓ HDL (<55 or 1.42 mmol/L) ↓ TSH (<2.0)
Thyroid hypofunction-primary	↑ TSH (>4.4) ↑ Triglycerides (>110 or 1.24 mmol/L) ↑ Cholesterol (>220 or 5.69mmol/L)	↓ T-3 (<100 or 1.54 nmol/L) ↓ T-4 (<6 or 7.2 nmol/L) ↓ T-3 uptake (<27)
Thyroid hypofunction-secondary due to anterior pituitary dysfunction	↑ Triglycerides (>110 or 1.24 mmol/L) ↑ Cholesterol (>220 or 5.69mmol/L) ↑ BUN (>16 or 5.71 mmol/L)	↓ TSH (<2.0) ↓ T-3 uptake (<27)
Tissue destruction	↑ Potassium (>4.5) ↑ LDH (>200) ↑ ESR (> 10 in ♀ and > 5 in ♂)	
Tissue inflammation/ destruction (GI, tendon/bursa, phlebitis, sinusitis, musculoskeletal)	↑ ESR (> 10 in ♀ and > 5 in ♂) ↑ Potassium (>4.5) ↑ Basophils ↑ ALP increased with liver, bone or gastric inflammation (>100)	
Urinary tract congestion	↑ Creatinine (>1.1 or 97.2 μmmol/dL) ↑ Monocytes (>7%)	

© Weatherby & Associates, LLC

CONDITION	HIGH	LOW
Vitamin B12/folate deficiency	↑ MCH (>31.9) ↑ MCV (>89.9) ↑ RDW (>13) ↑ Serum iron (>100 or >17.91 μmol/L) ↑ LDH (>200)	↓ RBCs (<3.9♀, <4.2♂) ↓ HCT (<37 or 0.37 in ♂ and <40 or 0.4 in ♂) ↓ HGB (<13.5 or 135 g/L in ♂ and <14 or 140 in ♂) ↓ Total WBC count (<5.0) ↓ Neutrophils (<40%) ↓ Uric acid (<3.5 or 208 μmol/dL)
Vitamin C need	↑ MCV (>89.9) ↑ Alk Phos (>100) ↑ Fibrinogen	↓ Albumin (<4.0 or 40 g/L) ↓ MCH (<28) ↓ MCHC (<32) ↓ HGB (<13.5 or 135 g/L in ♂ and <14 or 140 in ♂) ↓ HCT (<37 or 0.37 in ♂ and <40 or 0.4 in ♂) ↓ RBCs (<3.9♀, <4.2♂) ↓ Serum iron (<50 or <8.96 μmol/L)
Zinc deficiency		↓ Alkaline phosphatase (<70)

© Weatherby & Associates, LLC

www.BloodChemistryAnalysis.com

Discussion

The stained film examination provides information on red blood cell variation and abnormalities in red blood cell size, shape, hemoglobin content.

When would you run this test?

1. To help diagnose blood disorders: anemia, Thalassemia, and other hemoglobin disorders will have distinctive morphological changes that can be appreciated via a stained blood cell examination
2. As a guide to therapy: if therapy is effective the abnormalities will begin to clear up.
3. Often a Complete blood count (CBC) will include a stained red cell examination if gross abnormalities are seen

Clinical implications of abnormalities

Abnormality	Clinical Implication
Anisocytosis (abnormal variations in size)	Any severe anemia (iron deficiency, megaloblastic)
	Liver dysfunction
Microcytosis	Iron deficiency and iron loading anemia
	Thalassemia
	Lead poisoning
Macrocytosis	Megaloblastic anemia (Vitamin B12/foliate deficiency anemia)
	Liver disease
Macroovalocytosis	Megaloblastic anemia
Hypochromia (↓ concentration of hemoglobin)	Iron deficiency and iron loading anemia
	Thalassemia
	Lead poisoning
Nucleated red blood cells	Hemolytic anemia
	Leukemias
	Myeloproliferative diseases
	Multiple myeloma

Abnormality	Clinical Implication
Howell-Jolly bodies	✳ Hyposplenism
	✳ Pernicious anemia
Heinz bodies	✳ Congenital hemolytic anemias
	✳ Thalassemia
Siderocytes	✳ Iron loading anemia
	✳ Hyposplenism
	✳ Hemolytic anemia
Cabot's rings	✳ Pernicious anemia
	✳ Lead poisoning
Basophilic stippling	✳ Hemolytic anemia
	✳ Lead poisoning
Rouleaux	✳ Tissue hypoxia
	Ø Ph imbalances and dysbiosis
	Ø Poor protein metabolism
	Ø Liver dysfunction
	✳ Multiple myeloma
Poikilocytosis (abnormal variations in shape)	Ø Digestive disorders especially dysbiosis
	Ø Need for essential fatty acids
	Ø Increased free radical activity
	Ø Liver toxicity
	Ø Poor circulation
	✳ Any severe anemia

© Weatherby & Associates, LLC

Degree of Poikilocytosis

Certain shapes are diagnostically helpful. The following are shapes seen on stained blood examination:

Abnormality	Clinical Implication
Ovalocytes	Iron deficiency
	B12/folate imbalances
	Hormonal imbalance
Sickle cells	Sickle cell disease
Target cells	Liver disease and bile insufficiency
	Dysbiosis
	Iron deficiency
	Thalassemia
Shistocytes	Increased toxins
	Spleen dysfunction
	Uremia
Burr cells	Hemolytic anemias
	Liver disease
Acanthocytes	Liver and spleen dysfunction
	Ph and overall terrain imbalance
	Vitamin E deficiency
	Hypercholesterolemia
Teardrop cells	Lack of assimilation
	Liver dysfunction

TEST	REF. RANGE	RESULT	OPTIMAL ↓/↑
Glucose	65 – 115		80 – 100
HgB A1C	<7%		4.1 – 5.7%
BUN	5 – 25		10 – 16
Creatinine	0.6 – 1.5		0.8 – 1.1
Sodium	135 – 147		135 – 142
Potassium	3.5 – 5.3		4.0 – 4.5
Chloride	96 – 109		100 – 106
CO₂	22 – 32		25 – 30
Anion Gap	6 – 16		7 – 12
Uric Acid	2.2 – 7.7		3.5 – 5.9 male / 3.0 – 5.5 female
Total Protein	6.0 – 8.5		6.9 – 7.4
Albumin	3.5 – 5.5		4.0 – 5.0
Calcium	8.5 – 10.8		9.2 – 10.0
Phosphorous	2.5 – 4.5		3.0 – 4.0
Alk Phos	25 – 140		70 – 100
SGOT(AST)	0 – 40		10 – 30
SGPT(ALT)	0 – 45		10 – 30
LDH	1 – 240		140 – 200
total Bilirubin	0.1 – 1.2		0.1 – 1.2 (>2.6)
direct	0 – 0.2		0 – 0.2 (>0.8)
indirect	0.1 – 1.0		0.1 – 1.0 (>1.8)
GGTP	1 – 70		10 – 30
Globulin	2.0 – 3.9		2.4 – 2.8
A/G ratio	1.0 – 2.4		1.4 – 2.1
BUN/Creat.	7 – 18		10 – 16
Total iron	30 – 170		50 – 100
Cholesterol	130 – 200		150 – 220
Triglycerides	30 – 150		70 – 110
LDL	60 – 130		<120
HDL	40 – 90		>55
Chol/HDL	Ratio		<4
Ferritin	33 - 236		33 – 236 male / 10 – 122 female
	10 - 122		
TIBC	250 – 350		250 – 350
TSH	0.35 – 5.50		2.0 – 4.4
Free T-3	2.3 – 4.2		2.3 – 4.2
T-3	60 – 181		100 – 165
Free T-4	0.70 – 2.4		0.70 – 1.53
T-4 thyroxine	4.5 – 13.2		6 – 12
COMPLETE BLOOD COUNT			
WBC	3.7 – 10.5		5.0 – 7.5
RBC	4.1 – 5.6		4.2 – 4.9 male / 3.9 – 4.5 fem
	3.8 – 5.1		
Reticulocyte	0.5 – 1		0.5 – 1
Hemoglobin	12.5 – 17.0		14 – 15 male / 13.5 – 14.5 fem
	11.5 – 15.0		
Hematocrit	36 – 50%		40 – 48 male / 37 – 44 female
	34 – 44		
MCV	80 – 98		82 – 89.9
MCH	27 – 34		28 – 31.9
MCHC	32 – 36		32 – 35
Platelets	155 – 385		150 – 385 x 1000
RDW	11.7 – 15.0		<13
Neutrophils	40 – 74%		40 – 60%
Lymphs	14 – 46%		24 – 44%
Monocytes	4 – 13%		0 – 7%
Eosinophils	0 – 7%		0 – 3%
Basophils	0 – 3%		0 – 1%

NOTES

© Weatherby & Associates, LLC

CONVERSION CHART FOR CONVERTING STANDARD US UNITS INTO STANDARD INTERNATIONAL UNITS

TEST	US UNITS	CONVERSION FACTOR → Multiply ← Divide	S.I. UNITS
Glucose	mg/dL	0.05551	mmol/L
HgB A1C	%	0.01	
BUN	mg/dL	0.357	mmol/L
Creatinine	mg/dL	88.4	μmol/dL
Sodium	mEq/L	1	mmol/L
Potassium	mEq/L	1	mmol/L
Chloride	mEq/L	1	mmol/L
CO_2	mEq/L	1	mmol/L
Anion Gap	mEq/L	1	mmol/L
Uric Acid	mg/dL	59.48	μmol/dL
Total Protein	g/dL	10	g/L
Albumin	g/dL	10	g/L
Calcium	mg/dL	0.250	mmol/L
Phosphorous	mg/dL	0.3229	mmol/L
Alk Phos	U/L	1	U/L
SGOT(AST)	U/L	1	U/L
SGPT(ALT)	U/L	1	U/L
LDH	U/L	1	U/L
Bilirubin values	mg/dL	17.1	μmol/dL
GGTP	U/L	1	U/L
Globulin	g/dL	10	g/L
A/G ratio	Ratio	1	Ratio
BUN/Creat.	Ratio	1	Ratio
Total iron	mg/dL	0.1791	μmol/dL
Cholesterol	mg/dL	0.02586	mmol/L
Triglycerides	mg/dL	0.01129	mmol/L
LDL	mg/dL	0.02586	mmol/L
HDL	mg/dL	0.02586	mmol/L
Chol/HDL	Ratio	1	Ratio
Ferritin	ng/mL	1	μg/L
TIBC	μg/dL	0.1791	μmol/dL
TSH	μIU/mL	1	mIU/L
T-3 uptake	%	0.01	%
T-3	ng/dL	0.01536	nmol/L
Free T-3	pg/dl	0.01536	pmol/L
T-4 thyroxine	μg/dL	12.87	nmol/L
Free T-4	ng/dl	12.87	pmol/L
FTI/ T-7		1	
WBC	x 10^3/mm^3	1	10^9/L
RBC	x 10^6/mm^3	1	10^{12}/L
Hemoglobin	g/dL	10	g/L
Hematocrit	%	0.01	1
MCV	$Microns^3$	1	fL
MCH	pg	1	pg
MCHC	g/dL	1	1
Platelets	x 10^3/mm^3	1	10^9/L
RDW	Calculated	1	Calculated
Neutrophils	%	1	%
Lymphs	%	1	%
Monocytes	%	1	%
Eosinophils	%	1	%
Basophils	%	1	%

© Weatherby & Associates, LLC

CHEMSCREEN and CBC RESULTS TRACKING FORM STANDARD INTERNATIONAL UNITS

NAME: DATE:

TEST	REF. RANGE	RESULT	OPTIMAL	↓/↑
Glucose	3.61 – 6.38		4.44 – 5.55	
HgB A1C	<0.07		0.041 – 0.057	
BUN	1.79 – 8.93		3.57 – 5.71	
Creatinine	53.0 – 132.6		70.7 – 97.2	
Sodium	135 – 147		135 – 142	
Potassium	3.5 – 5.3		4.0 – 4.5	
Chloride	96 – 109		100 – 106	
CO_2	22 – 32		25 – 30	
Anion Gap	6 – 16		7 – 12	
Uric Acid	131 – 458		208 – 351 male 178 – 327 female	
Total Protein	60 – 85		69 – 74	
Albumin	35 – 55		40 – 50	
Calcium	2.13 – 2.70		2.30 – 2.50	
Phosphorous	0.81 – 1.45		0.97 – 1.29	
Alk Phos	25 – 140		70 – 100	
SGOT(AST)	0 – 40		10 – 30	
SGPT(ALT)	0 – 45		10 – 30	
LDH	1 – 240		140 – 200	
total Bilirubin	1.7 – 20.5		1.7 – 20.5 (>44.5)	
direct	0 – 3.4		0 – 3.4 (>13.7)	
indirect	1.7 – 17.1		1.7 – 17.1 (>30.8)	
GGTP	1 – 70		10 – 30	
Globulin	20 – 39		24 – 28	
A/G ratio	1.1 – 2.5		1.5 – 2.0	
BUN/Creat.	7 – 14		13 – 17	
Total iron	5.37 – 30.45		8.96 – 17.91	
Cholesterol	3.36 – 5.20		3.9 – 5.69	
Triglycerides	0.34 – 1.7		0.79 – 1.24	
LDL	1.55 – 3.36		<3.1	
HDL	1.03 – 2.32		>1.42	
Chol/HDL	Ratio		<4	
Ferritin	33 - 236 10 - 122		33 – 236 male 10 – 122 female	
TIBC	44.8 – 62.7		44.8 – 62.7	
TSH	0.35 – 5.50		2.0 – 4.4	
Free T-3	3.59 – 6.56		3.59 – 6.56	
T-3	1.23 – 3.53		1.54 – 3.53	
Free T4	9.1 – 31.0		9.1 – 19.7	
T-4 thyroxine	61.8 – 169.9		77.2 – 154.4	
COMPLETE BLOOD COUNT				
WBC	3.7 – 10.5		5.0 – 7.5	
RBC	4.1 – 5.6 3.8 – 5.1		4.2 – 4.9 male 3.9 – 4.5 fem	
Reticulocyte	0.5 – 1		0.5 – 1	
Hemoglobin	125 – 170 115 – 150		140 – 150 male 135 – 145 fem	
Hematocrit	0.36 – 0.50 0.34 – 0.44		0.40 – 0.48 male 0.37 – 0.44 fem	
MCV	80 – 98		82 – 89.9	
MCH	27 – 34		28 – 31.9	
MCHC	32 – 36		32 – 35	
Platelets	155 – 385		150 – 385 x 1000	
RDW	11.7 – 15.0		<13	
Neutrophils	40 – 74%		40 – 60%	
Lymphs	14 – 46%		24 – 44%	
Monocytes	4 – 13%		0 – 7%	
Eosinophils	0 – 7%		0 – 3%	
Basophils	0 – 3%		0 – 1%	

NOTES

© Weatherby & Associates, LLC

www.BloodChemistryAnalysis.com

The "Four Quadrants of Functional Diagnosis"
Diagnostic Education for the *Functional Age*

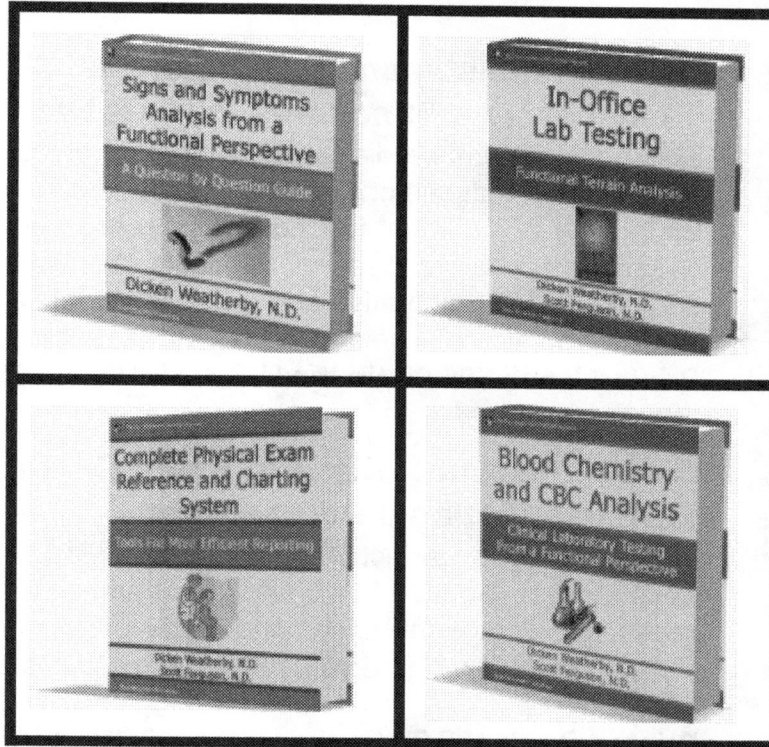

Most of us at some point or other have come to recognize that the diagnostic tests we learned in medical school taught us nothing about how to uncover our patients' functional problems. This is why I wrote my first book, *"Blood Chemistry and CBC Analysis- Clinical Laboratory Testing From a Functional Perspective"* with my colleague Dr. Scott Ferguson, to make the wealth of functional information you can get from a standard Chemistry Screen and CBC available to health care practitioners. This book and other products in my "Four Quadrants of Functional Diagnosis" series are designed to give you and your practice the same functional diagnostic education that thousands of practitioners have been using successfully in their practices.

The *Four Quadrants of Functional Diagnosis* will help you:
- Get excellent patient results
- Dramatically improve your clinical outcomes
- Get more referrals
- Cut the amount of time you spend analyzing your patient cases
- Set up a system of functional tests that will be the envy of all your colleagues

In preparing for the Functional Age, the rules on how to manage the diagnostic information in your practice have changed. You can no longer blindly use the same tests every one else is using and hope to get different results. The Functional Age will require that you have more information to be able to properly find the cause of your patients' problems. *Signs and Symptoms Analysis from A Functional Perspective, Boost Clinic Income With an In-Office Lab System,* and *The Functional Blood Chemistry Analysis System* were developed for practitioners just like you who recognize the need for a new paradigm in diagnostic information. Practitioners who realize that the Pathological Age is over and the Functional Age has begun.

Dr. Dicken Weatherby, Naturopathic Physician

Functional Blood Chemistry Analysis

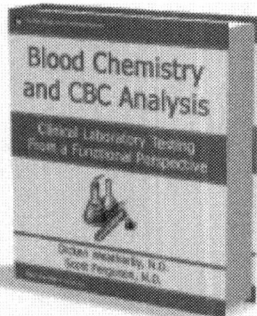

Blood Chemistry and CBC Analysis- Clinical Laboratory Testing from a Functional Perspective

This book presents a diagnostic system of blood chemistry and CBC analysis that focuses on physiological function as a marker of health. By looking for optimum function we increase our ability to detect dysfunction long before disease manifests. Conventional lab testing becomes a truly preventative and prognostic tool. A must for any practitioners who wants to get more from the tests they are already running.
Printed Book $65.00 (in the U.S.A.) ISBN: 0-9761367-1-6

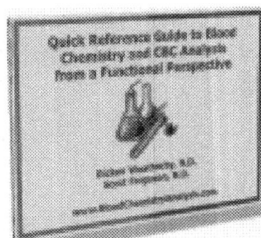

Quick Reference Guide to Blood Chemistry Analysis From a Functional Perspective

This guide is the perfect companion to our Blood Chemistry and CBC Analysis Book. It is a complete reference for interpreting, analyzing, and finding the underlying cause of your patients' functional complaints. You will find yourself referring to this guide over and over again.
Printed Book $35.00 (in the U.S.A.) ISBN: 0-9761367-8-3

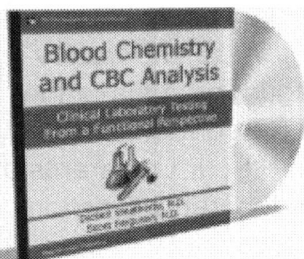

Functional Blood Chemistry Analysis Seminar on Audio

Any practitioners of the healing arts will gain a tremendous benefit from listening to this complete one day seminar on audio CD. Dr. Weatherby guides the listener through his method of analyzing blood chemistry and CBC tests. Topics include using standard blood tests to analyze the following: GI dysfunction, minerals and vitamin insufficiencies, blood sugar dysregulation, cardiovascular problems, thyroid issues, and adrenal dysfunction..
6 hours of audio $147.00 (in the U.S.A.) ISBN: 0-9726469-4-9

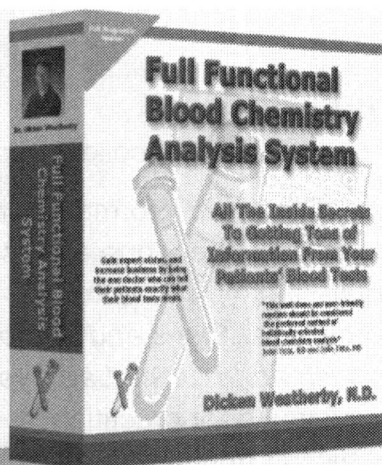

The Full Functional Blood Chemistry Analysis System is a complete road map to success that shows you exactly how to approach each blood chemistry analysis step by step. This system includes the printed reference book, the Quick Reference Guide, and the Audio Recordings, a system for getting the most out of your blood chemistry tests.

A functional diagnosis of your patients' blood test results is one of the most effective diagnostic tools to get to the bottom of the myriad of health complaints your patients present with. Gain expert status, and increase business by being the one doctor who can tell patients exactly what their blood tests mean.
Full Blood Chemistry System $197.00 (in the U.S.A.) ISBN: 0-9761367-3-2

In-Office Lab Testing
Boost Your Clinic Income!

I want you to be successful in your practice and to have the same tools that I use to increase clinical efficacy and clinic income, which is why I created my *Boost Clinic Income With an In-Office Lab System*. The tests I present in this system will help you get a wealth of functional data from your patients and the income you make on these tests stays in your practice. At the heart of this system is my Functional Urinalysis program.

Functional Urinalysis allows you to run a series of simple urine tests that get to the heart of the disturbances in your patients' inner "terrain". These tests have been used for many years but until now the interpretive information available to health care practitioners has been poor. I have put together the most comprehensive system for understanding and interpreting the Functional Urinalysis. Watch the instructional DVD, listen to the 2 audio CDs packed with time saving tips and interpretive tools, refer to the in-depth reference manual, and start paying for your office overhead with Functional Urinalysis!

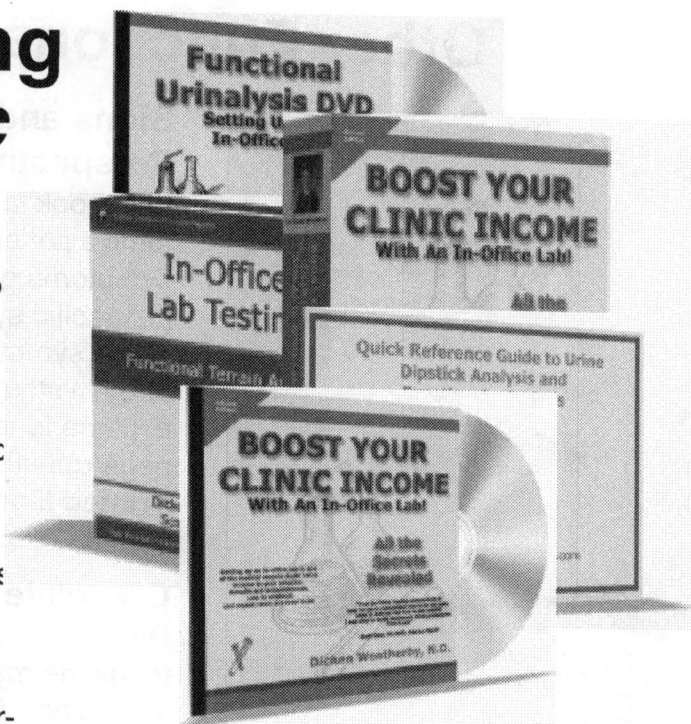

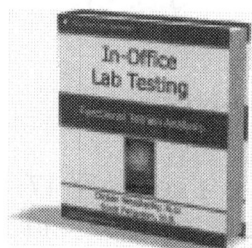

Reference Manual
$85.00 (in the U.S.A)
ISBN: 0-9761367-4-0

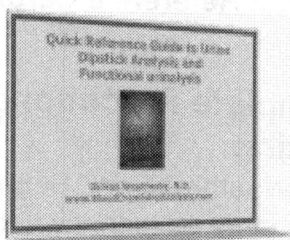

Urine Dipstick Guide
$35.00 (in the U.S.A)
ISBN: 0-9761367-9-1

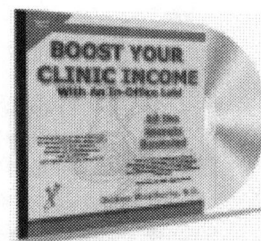

**Functional Urinalysis
Audio Program**
$85.00 (in the U.S.A)

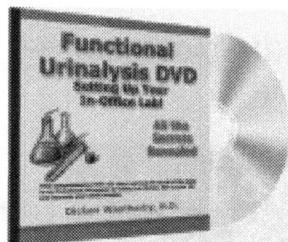

Functional Urinalysis DVD
$85.00 (in the U.S.A)

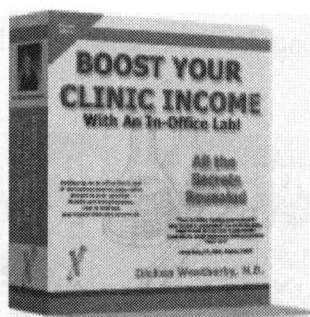

Get the complete **"Boost Clinic Income With an In-Office Lab"** system to rapidly increase your clinic income with Functional Urinalysis and other in-office labs. Save $43.00 by getting all the above tools bundled together. **$247.00 (in the U.S.A)**
ISBN: 09726469-1-4

Other Functional Diagnostic Tools

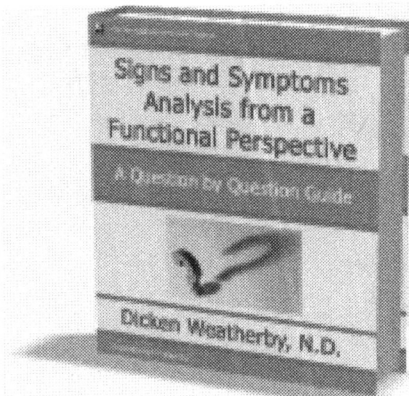

Signs and Symptoms Analysis From a Functional Perspective

This book takes a critical look at the myriad of signs and symptoms a patient presents with. Using a comprehensive signs and symptoms questionnaire you can look at the symptom burden in specific systems of the body, address some of the more obscure symptoms, and track changes over time. Organized by body systems, this book provides the nutritional and functional explanations behind the 322 questions on Dr. Weatherby's 4-page questionnaire.

Printed Book $65.00 (in the U.S.A.) ISBN: 0-9761367-2-4

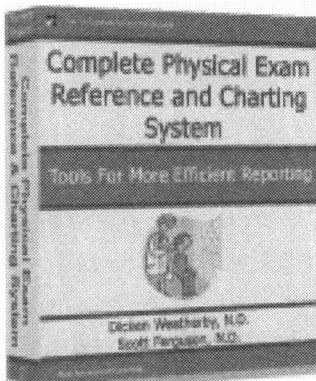

Complete PE Reference and Charting System

Drs. Weatherby and Ferguson have put together report forms for all the major physical examinations commonly performed in your office (i.e. cardiovascular, lung, abdominal, neurological examinations). These report forms provide an easy method of charting and filing your physical examination results.

The accompanying reference cards fit neatly into your white coat and provide a detailed explanation of all the tests on each report form and are an excellent "exam-side" reference to refresh your memory on all the different tests that make up each examination.

Printed Reference Cards and CD $65.00 (in the U.S.A.)

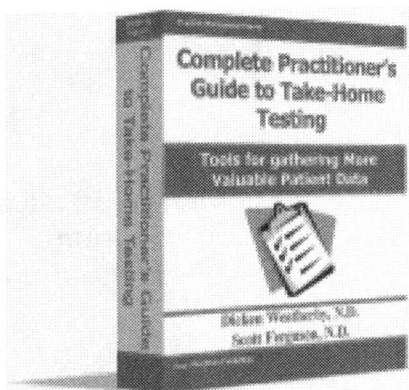

Complete Practitioner's Guide to Take-Home Testing

Drs. Weatherby and Ferguson have put together a series of 17 take-home tests that you can give to your patients to perform in between their office visits. These tests will allow you to assess for digestion, elimination, zinc status, pH regulation, hypothyroid conditions, iodine insufficiency, blood type, and food and other sensitivities and intolerances. Patient "homework" is an important method of gathering patient data and encouraging compliance.

Printed Book $45.00 (in the U.S.A.) ISBN: 0-9761367-7-5

**To Order Any Functional Diagnostic Product
Please Visit Our Website
www.BloodChemistryAnalysis.com**

Quick Order Form

Fax Orders: 541-899-6854. Send this form.

Telephone orders: Call 541-899-1522

Email orders: orders@BloodChemistryAnalysis.com

Secure online orders: http://www.BloodChemistryAnalysis.com/diagnosisshop.html

Postal orders: Bear Mountain Publishing, 7000 Little Applegate Road, Jacksonville, OR 97530, USA. Telephone: 541-899-1522

Please send the following books, CDs or reports. I understand that I may return any of them for a full refund – for any reason, no questions asked.

_____
_____
_____

Please send more FREE information on:

☐ Other books   ☐ Live Seminars or Teleseminars   ☐ Speaking   ☐ Consulting

Name:_____

Address:_____

City:_____ State: _____ Zip:_____

Phone:_____ E-mail:_____

Shipping by air
US: $4.00 for first book and $2.00 for each additional product.
International: $9.00 for first book; $5.00 for each additional product (estimate)

Payment: ☐ Cheque   ☐ Credit Card

☐ Visa   ☐ Mastercard   ☐ AMEX   ☐ Discover

Personal check (payable to Bear Mountain Publishing):

Card number:_____

Name on card:_____Exp. Date:_____

http://www.BloodChemistryAnalysis.com

www.ingramcontent.com/pod-product-compliance
Lightning Source LLC
Chambersburg PA
CBHW082113210326
41599CB00033B/6686